Neuropathy

How to Effectively Treat Peripheral Neuropathy

(Simple Ways to Stop Diabetic Neuropathy & Get Your Health Back)

Melissa Reed

Published By **Regina Loviusher**

Melissa Reed

Neuropathy: How to Effectively Treat Peripheral Neuropathy (Simple Ways to Stop Diabetic Neuropathy & Get Your Health Back)

ISBN   978-1-998769-46-9

No part of this guidebook shall be reproduced in any form without permission in writing from the publisher except in the case of brief quotations embodied in critical articles or reviews.

Legal & Disclaimer

The information contained in this ebook is not designed to replace or take the place of any form of medicine or professional medical advice. The information in this ebook has been provided for educational & entertainment purposes only.

The information contained in this book has been compiled from sources deemed reliable, and it is accurate to the best of the Author's knowledge; however, the Author cannot guarantee its accuracy and validity and cannot be held liable for any errors or omissions. Changes are periodically made to this book. You must consult your doctor or get professional medical advice before using any of the suggested remedies, techniques, or information in this book.

Upon using the information contained in this book, you agree to hold harmless the Author from and against any damages, costs, and expenses, including any legal fees potentially resulting from the application of any of the information provided by this guide. This disclaimer applies to any damages or injury caused by the use and application, whether directly or indirectly, of any advice or information presented, whether for breach of contract, tort, negligence, personal injury, criminal intent, or under any other cause of action.

You agree to accept all risks of using the information presented inside this book. You need to consult a professional medical practitioner in order to ensure you are both able and healthy enough to participate in this program.

Table Of Contents

Chapter 1: What Is Neuropathy?.............. 1

Chapter 2: The Different Types Of
Neuropathy... 4

Chapter 3: The Symptoms Of Neuropathy
In Feet.. 8

Chapter 4: The Serious Effects Of
Neuropathy... 14

Chapter 5: How Neuropathy Leads To
Social Exclusion..................................... 19

Chapter 6: Diabetes And Neuropathy 24

Chapter 7: Causes Of Diabetic Neuropathy
.... 31

Chapter 8: Peripheral Neuropathy
Treatment... 37

Chapter 9: Natural Approaches To Cope
With Diabetic Neuropathy 41

Chapter 10: Neuropathy Therapy Options
That Can Keep You Moving 46

Chapter 11: Reducing Neuropathy The Natural Way... 50

Chapter 12: Nutrition's Role In Neuropathy 54

Chapter 13: Reversing Neuropathy 60

Chapter 14: Peripheral Neuropathy Symptoms.. 64

Chapter 15: How To Manage Neuropathy 69

Chapter 16: Keys To Effective Neuropathy Treatment.. 73

Chapter 17: Getting Positive About Your Neuropathy Treatment 78

Chapter 18: Pain Management And Neuropathy Therapy 82

Chapter 19: How To Get Maximum Benefits From Acupuncture Treatment For Neuropathy... 86

Chapter 20: Habits And Routines: Powerful Neuropathy Treatment Weapons 94

Chapter 1: What Is Neuropathy?

What is neuropathy? Why is it becoming such a threat? Why do people fear it? Unfortunately, it's because of the 'hard-to-detect' nature of peripheral neuropathy that makes it such as dangerous condition.

You may not know but you already have it. Its symptoms are usually harmless and can occur with any person. One minute, they'll feel a small tingling sensation in their foot, the next it had already spread throughout their bodies.

Neuropathy, in simple definition, is actually nerve damage. Because the blood does not circulate the right way, the nerve underneath the skin do not receive the right amount of oxygen it needs to function. More often than note, the feet are the ones that are first to be affected.

It is also a body part that usually experiences occasional numbness or pain due to footwear, external conditions and so on. Apart from neuropathy in feet and hands, it can also occur with organs and senses. People have lost the ability to sense temperature and even to see or hear because of different kinds of neuropathy.

Yet another fact that makes neuropathy dangerous is that doctors haven't found a way to heal it. Many experts and groups claim that herbs and traditional medicine work on this but these are yet to be proven.

In addition to this, scientists have conducted numerous experiments with magnets or infrared lights. Most of these have been proven effective in treating nerve damage temporarily. Bottom line is that neuropathy has no permanent cure as of now.

However, even with these, neuropathy can still be prevented. Some of the major causes for neuropathy are sicknesses such as diabetes or poor eating habits. By focusing on a healthy lifestyle, you'll be able to avoid these.

Food and exercise are great factors in preventing peripheral neuropathy. This way, neuropathy may be a threat but there will always be a way to defend against it.

Chapter 2: The Different Types Of Neuropathy

Neuropathy, also known as peripheral neuropathy, is a disease often associated with diabetes, although there are actually more than 100 known types of the disease - each with its own characteristic symptoms, pattern of development, and prognosis.

Although there are several "tell-tale" symptoms that seem to afflict all neuropathy sufferers, each version of the disease is different and comes with its own set of problems.

Below are several of the main types of neuropathy, although this is not an exhaustive listing by any means.

Diabetic neuropathy - Over 30% of all neuropathies can be linked to diabetes, and diabetes is the most common cause of neuropathy in the western world. Both Type 1 and Type 2 diabetes can lead to diabetic neuropathy - high blood sugar levels damage the nerves and neuropathy is one of the outcomes.

Immune Mediated/CIDP - manifestations of neuropathy such as CIDP (Chronic Inflammatory Demyelinating Polyneuropathy) is caused by an abnormal immune system response.

In this condition, nerves swell and become irritated due to an immune reaction, eventually damaging the nerves outside the brain or spinal cord with peripheral neuropathy symptoms thus following.

Hereditary neuropathy - Diseases like Charcot-Marie-Tooth have been discovered to be inherited and lead to hereditary neuropathy. This condition deals with the role of different proteins in the role of physiology in peripheral nerve conduction.

Autonomic neuropathy - actually a group of symptoms more than a disease itself, autonomic neuropathy concerns damage to the nerves of the body that control every-day functions in the body that are autonomic in nature, such as blood pressure, heart rate, bowel and bladder emptying, even digestion.

When the nerves that control or affect these functions are disrupted, these autonomic functions cease to perform normally and can cause many complications.

Compressive neuropathy - Known to laymen as a "pinched nerve," compressive neuropathy often comes about by an accidental injury to the body. Herniated discs, sciatica, arthritis in the spine and spinal stenosis are just some of the ways a nerve can become compressed and cause pain and discomfort to an afflicted sufferer.

Drug-Induced/Toxic neuropathy - toxic polyneuropathies come about in the human body when nerves are damaged or destroyed by chemicals introduced that have cumulative or highly-toxic effects. These tend to be occupational, chance exposures or intentional, even homicidal ingestions.

There are other forms of neuropathy, including those from infectious diseases such as shingles, as well as from nutritional deficiencies. The best bet for understanding any form of neuropathy that a person may be experiencing is to visit their doctor or a trained neurologist for a consultation.

Chapter 3: The Symptoms Of Neuropathy In Feet

Peripheral neuropathy and diabetic neuropathy are associated with nerve damage that can translate to nerve problems all over the body, including the feet.

Neuropathy in feet is a particularly nasty condition that can leave the sufferer in agony, or lead to amputation. Also, neuropathy in feet can be caused by nerve damage that results from disease and conditions, such as: HIV/AIDS, diabetes, alcoholism, and Lyme disease.

Common Symptoms of Neuropathy in Feet

The most common symptoms of foot neuropathy are: tingling feet, numb feet, and foot pain that can radiate up the foot and into the legs. The tingling and numbness are caused by the misfiring of the damaged nerves in the feet and the peripheral nervous system.

Advanced Symptoms of Neuropathy

As the disease progresses the symptoms will become steadily worse. The pain will become sharper, and the tingling sensations will become more like electrical shocks.

Also, some sufferers will experience a burning sensation in their feet. These symptoms can be relieved using topical creams, but most people find pain relief when using therapies, such as acupuncture and massage therapy.

Severe Symptoms of Neuropathy

The longer the condition is present the worse the symptoms. As the nerve damage becomes more severe, the sufferer will begin to notice that the pain is unbearable, or that the numbness has spread and become more pronounced. This numbness can be dangerous, because lack of sensation in the feet can lead to loss of balance.

Once the condition has progressed this far, topical neuropathy creams, acupuncture and massage therapy may no longer be effective neuropathy treatments, but you may find success using nerve support formula, which is an herbal supplement that can help improve nerve function.

Neuropathy in feet is a potentially dangerous condition that has many treatments, but no cure. Visit your physician often to learn about the newest and most effective neuropathy treatments available. Keeping ahead of the neuropathy treatment game will help you find pain relief despite the severity of your neuropathy.

The symptoms of neuropathy in feet can be varied but treatment options are almost always available. For a free trial of a clinically proven treatment option, visit Treating Neuropathy in Feet

In general, neuropathy symptoms begin with lack of sensation, prickling in the toes or fingers, and continue to extend to the feet and hands, causing burning sensation and severe pain, which is particularly acute at night time.

Neuropathy pain is usually symmetrical, meaning one would have the pain on both sides of the body -on both feet and both hands, for example. Peripheral neuropathy usually develops suddenly.

Symptoms include numbness, where patients feel as if they are wearing invisible gloves, acute pain, excessive sensitivity to pain, muscle weakness, loss of balance, high or low blood pressure, trouble with moving muscles, lack of sleep due to pain, and atypical sweating.

The type of symptom of peripheral neuropathy depends on the nerves that are damaged, and this depends on the origin of the disease. Two causes of neuropathy are diabetes and alcoholism.

Symptoms for diabetic neuropathy include numbness, tickling or pricking pain. Some cases of diabetic neuropathy show no symptoms at all, while others can be so sudden, that they cause immediate disability.

The pain may be either unbearable, or cause insensitivity to any kind of pain, both of which are dangerous.

Neuropathy pain may also be mild at the start and go unnoticed, but over a period of time, it could become severe and complicated. Diabetic neuropathy could cause urinary and gastrointestinal problems, weakness, and problems with sexual organs.

Symptoms for alcoholic neuropathy include sharp pains, lack of sensation, urinary control, feeling like the bladder is not completely empty, problems with starting to urinate, muscle spasms, lack of ability to tolerate normal body heat, nausea, constipation and impotence.

Other notable symptoms can be drooping eyelids, varying tone of voice while speaking, difficulty with swallowing, and problems with speech itself in some cases.

Neuropathic pain may be sudden or gradual; it manifests in different ways, depending on its origin (such as with diabetes or alcoholism). What is common to all neuropathy, however, is the danger to and the suffering of the patient, who ought to seek treatment as soon as they are aware of the problem.

Chapter 4: The Serious Effects Of Neuropathy

Usually peripheral neuropathy strikes those people who are diabetic and not seriously concerned about the disorder until the condition worsens and severe symptoms start to manifest.

Because the nerve signals are disrupted due to damage in the nerves, peripheral neuropathy ensues. The warning signs range from tingling sensations to jabbing and sharp electric pain in the patient's extremities.

They are usually manifested in the hands and feet of the person with neuropathy. The indicators differ from one person to another and depend on the stage of the disorder. Coordination and synchronization between the body parts are affected and so is mobility.

Thus, a person with neuropathy will find it very difficult to complete his daily responsibilities and will become weak since the symptoms of this disorder are terribly depressing and can make a person feel low and despondent in most cases.

A reality to be accepted about neuropathy

One of the major setbacks of this disorder is that the condition cannot be reversed. Medications and home treatments can only reduce the pain and alleviate the symptoms and slow the advancement of further damage.

People with peripheral neuropathy often feel as if they are wearing gloves and socks since the sensations in their feet and hands are usually completely annulled for them to feel anything.

How would you feel knowing that the only direction you can go with your condition is forward. This is why it is strongly suggested for medical practitioners to carefully set expectations of neuropathy patients.

Giving them false hopes will only have a boomerang effect on both of you. Emphasis must be put on the need to cope with the condition and not entirely on curing it.

It is mandatory for diabetic patients to have their routine check-up done in a regular basis. Diabetics must closely monitor and keep their blood glucose levels within normal range.

Untreated increase of blood sugar level creates a hazardous scenario for diabetic individuals. In addition, one's lifestyle has to be modified in such a way that it would promote wellness rather than complication of symptoms.

Included in such modifications would be proper and regular hygiene, skin and wound care, and proper diet and eating habits. Diabetics should take extra care of their feet because peripheral neuropathy is usually detected in the feet.

With proper guidance and medication early detection of neuropathy will prevent it from progressing further. Life can still be worth-living as long as you get to cope with neuropathy.

Chapter 5: How Neuropathy Leads To Social Exclusion

Neuropathy sometimes can be severely debilitating and may adversely affect a person's social life. It may seriously limit a person's functioning and may make even everyday simple tasks almost impossible to complete.

Certain severe forms of neuropathy like the Guillain-Barre Syndrome may make a person completely bedridden for many weeks, while in many other cases, like autonomic neuropathy causing incontinence, the affected person voluntarily starts avoiding all social gatherings due to fear of embarrassment.

Neuropathy may cause social exclusion by severely disabling a person. Often patients with neuropathy may have difficulty in walking and sometimes even frank ataxia also. Patients might develop certain deformities, for example, claw hand due to nerve damage, and may start avoiding social gatherings.

The pain and altered sensations like tingling, numbness and other paraesthesias associated with neuropathy sometimes might be very severe and may make the patient seek comfort of home more rather than going out. Diabetic patients with distal neuropathy affecting the lower limbs may prefer to stay at home due to fear of causing injury to the foot.

Diabetes often runs in families, and many a times, the patients have witnessed in other family members the serious complications arising from such an injury and are thus are very cautious. Bowel disturbances like severe diarrhea may also make a person more and more confined to home, especially if he has other symptoms of neuropathy.

One way in which involvement of autonomic nervous system in neuropathy may present is with incontinence. The most common form is urinary incontinence but fecal incontinence may also occur. In urinary incontinence, there is involuntary leakage of urine from the bladder.

Similarly, in fecal incontinence, there is an involuntary passage of stool. Incontinence is one of the most important causes of social exclusion in people suffering from neuropathy. The social withdrawal is most often voluntary due to fear of humiliation and embarrassment.

Patients tend to avoid all social gatherings and prefer to remain confined to their homes. Autonomic neuropathy may also cause impotence in men and make them socially withdrawn because of low self-esteem because of being unable to achieve erection.

Sometimes autonomic neuropathy may present as gustatory sweating, in which there is profuse sweating on forehead, face, scalp and neck whenever a person ingests food.

A person may feel very embarrassed by this condition and may start becoming socially withdrawn due to fear of embarrassment. These are few examples of how a neuropathy can lead to social exclusion.

Chapter 6: Diabetes And Neuropathy

Neuropathies are a variety of ailments which arise when nerves of the peripheral nervous system - the nervous system aside from the brain and spinal cord - are damaged; this is most commonly referred to as peripheral neuropathy. Approximately 50% to 70% of the people who suffer with diabetes, in all probability will have some form of neuropathy.

Most often it affects the motor nerves which control muscle movement and the sensory nerves which are responsible for our awareness of sensations such as coldness or pain. It first becomes apparent in the extremities but can manifest itself in the heart, blood vessels, bladder and intestines

Types of Diabetic Neuropathy

Diabetic Neuropathy is often classified into four distinct categories: peripheral, autonomic, proximal and focal. Since neuropathy can affect nerves throughout the body this classification is dependent on which part of the body is affected.

(a) Peripheral neuropathy is the most common type and causes loss of feeling or pain in the hands, arms, toes, feet and legs. It can also cause muscle weakness and foot deformities. Due to the loss of feeling, injuries can go unnoticed, resulting in infection(s) and additional complications.

(b) Autonomic neuropathy affects the nerves which support the heart and blood vessels, the urinary tract, the lungs and eyes, the sex organs, the sweat glands and the digestive system. Autonomic neuropathy can also be responsible for hypoglycemia unawareness whereby a person no longer experience the warning symptoms of low blood sugar levels.

(c) Proximal neuropathy affects the thighs, hips, or buttocks resulting in weakness of the legs. Due to weakness of the legs it becomes difficult to go from a sitting to standing position and assistance may be required. This affliction is more common among persons with Type 2 diabetes.

(d) Focal neuropathy affects one nerve or a group of nerves leading to muscle weakness or pain. It can affect the nerves which control the facial muscles, eyes, ears, chest, abdomen, pelvis and lower back, thighs, legs and feet. It is painful and unpredictable, existing mostly among older adults suffering with diabetes. It tends to improve by itself and does not cause long-term damage.

Symptoms

The symptoms are dependent on: the type of neuropathy contracted, the nerve(s) affected (autonomic, motor, sensory) and their location. It is not uncommon for many types of neuropathy to affect all three types of nerves. Some neuropathies may appear suddenly while others develop gradually.

(a) Autonomic Nerve Damage: Swollen abdomen, Blurred vision, Feeling full quickly, Nausea/ Vomiting after eating, Constipation, Diarrhoea, Weight loss, Dizziness/Fainting, Overflow and/or Urinary incontinence, Difficulty beginning to urinate, Abnormal perspiring, Sensitivity to heat, Impotence in men and Vaginal dryness in women.

(b) Motor Nerve Damage: Experiencing difficulty to move a part of the body (loss of balance and coordination), Lack of dexterity and muscle control, Cramps or Spasms, Loss of muscle tissue and difficulty swallowing or breathing.

(c) Sensory Nerve Damage: Nerve pain, Tingling or numbness, Burning sensations, Lack of coordination and a Lessening or absence of sensation to such an extent that nothing can be felt.

Prevention Is Better Than Cure

Presently there's no cure for diabetic neuropathy. Treatments are focused on prevention of further damage to the nerves and relief of pain (to those already afflicted) and are often determined by the extent to which the ailment has progressed.

Antidepressants (low doses), Analgesics and anticonvulsant drugs may be prescribed for relief of burning, tingling and pain. Pills, creams, special diets and therapies to stimulate the nerves and muscles are also employed. Non-medicinal therapies may include: meditation, yoga, acupuncture, chiropractic massages and cognitive therapy. All treatments depend on the type of nerve problem and symptom.

Good foot health is particularly important and special preventative steps should be taken to avoid degenerative progress of the disease:

(a) Avoid continuous pressure on the knees and elbows

(b) Do not walk barefooted

(c) Avoid getting your feet too hot or cold

(d) Wash your feet daily with lukewarm water and mild soap

(e) Dry your feet well and use non-medicated powders with shoes, socks and stockings

(f) Apply cream or lotion to keep foot, especially heels smooth.

(g) Daily foot exams, checking for cuts, blisters, calluses or bruises.

The best way of preventing diabetic neuropathy is by adhering to the recommended treatment for your diabetes as prescribed by your doctor.

Taking your diabetes medicines or insulin, blood glucose monitoring, a proper diet and physical activity will help keep your blood sugar levels under control. Keeping your blood glucose level as close to normal as possible will help protect the nerves throughout the entire body.

Chapter 7: Causes Of Diabetic Neuropathy

If you are a diabetic then you should realize the importance of strictly monitoring your blood sugar levels and taking all possible action to keep it within the prescribed range.

Several complications including diabetic neuropathy, diabetic retinopathy, glaucoma and cataracts can quickly join diabetes in causing further harm to your body. Here are some different causes of diabetic neuropathy and some steps that can be taken by you to remain in control of the disease.

In addition to regular monitoring and delivery of insulin, you will also need to maintain a strict control over your diet and also exercise regularly to increase your body's metabolism and improve your blood circulation.

Diabetics suffer from poor blood circulation and nerve end damage due to uncontrolled blood sugar levels. Hence if your blood glucose fluctuates wildly or if you have had diabetes for a longer period of time then you could develop diabetic neuropathy.

If you are obese and have not given up smoking or drinking, then that too could lead you towards the path of diabetic neuropathy. If you had any injury to your nerves or suffer from inflammation of the nerves, or lastly get caught in the heredity trap, then that too could add another cause for diabetic neuropathy.

In other words diabetic neuropathy hinders the nerves ability to transmit signals from the brain and can also damage blood vessels that transport vital nutrients and oxygen to nerves.

Diabetic neuropathy itself is classified into 4 groups. The first one is Autonomic neuropathy which affects digestion, bladder and bowel movements and also impairs sexual functions. It can also affect nerves leading to the heart, eyes and lungs.

The second is Peripheral neuropathy which affects the movement and feelings in hands, legs, feet and toes. The third type is Focal neuropathy in which any nerve or a group of nerves in the body experiences abrupt pain or weakness.

The fourth type is proximal neuropathy which can cause pain in the buttocks, hips or thighs, which in turn can lead to weakness in the legs. Unfortunately you will not realize which diabetic neuropathy is going to attack your body until you start exhibiting the symptoms.

You should not ignore your problems and rush to your doctor at a late stage, but instead rush immediately so that you can be put on medications in a bid to slow down the effects of diabetic neuropathy. You can even go in for surgery in case you suffer from diabetic retinopathy.

There are also alternative natural treatments available in the form of antioxidants such as alpha lipoic acid capsules, which can lessen the pain associated with diabetic neuropathy and can also help to balance blood glucose levels

These capsules can also help in the treatment of diabetic pets such as dogs and horses but cannot be used on cats due to a toxic reaction with its liver. One simple method to stay ahead of diabetic neuropathy is regular examinations at hospitals or at your doctor's clinic.

A healthy diet and regular exercise to build up vital muscle tissue can also go a long way in delaying or avoiding this unwanted complication associated with diabetes.

Hence, even though diabetes brings along its own baggage of associated complications, you can still beat them with diet, exercise and regular tests. Pay heed to the different causes of diabetic neuropathy and discontinue any bad habits that could hasten the onset of the disease.

Chapter 8: Peripheral Neuropathy Treatment

A body can encounter trauma resulting in peripheral neuropathy which simply stated means damage to the nervous system. When damage or trauma has been had to the nerve cells the body undergoes a lack of feeling and sensations where the trauma has occurred.This disease is a heartbreaking one that can leave a person struggling to control the obsessive tingling in their feet and numbness in their hands.

Once thought to be a life changing and crippling disease, research regarding peripheral neuropathy has shown there are steps to overcoming the painful symptoms that comes with this painful diagnosis.

A Healthy lifestyle

A healthy diet and lifestyle not only promotes good health but for those who have been diagnosed with diabetes maintain a healthy weight and regular exercise can prevent the onset of diabetic neuropathy. Selecting a healthy diet that is rich in antioxidants, low in fat and high in protein will help a diabetic reduce his or her chances of developing neuropathy in feet.

Avoiding Hazards

Peripheral neuropathy can be developed sue to hazards that could have been avoided to some degree. Poisonous toxins such as alcohol, drugs and over usage of the vitamin B6 can lead to neuropathy when it could have been avoided.

Manage the pain

Pain relief for tingling feet and numb feet is possible with some neuropathy treatment. Topical creams are available to help lessen the pain for a period of time as well as taking some form of prescribed medication has proven to be somewhat effective for short term relief.

Recent research has shown that a combination of vitamins, herbs, and Alpha-Lipoic can actually help restore the nerve damage and give longer lasting pain relief.

Peripheral neuropathy treatments are available you just need to explore your options and discover which treatment works best for you.

Getting back to an active life

Just because you have been diagnosed with peripheral neuropathy does not mean your life is over and must end with this horrible bit of news.

You can choose to embrace the diagnosis research treatment options and then get back to the active life you enjoyed before the pain took its toll. Getting out and being active will only promote good health as you use your muscles and regain your movement.

Chapter 9: Natural Approaches To Cope With Diabetic Neuropathy

Diabetic neuropathy is a condition characterized by nerve damage in feet as a result of a long history of diabetes. Neuropathy in feet and hands usually develops in patients with poorly controlled blood sugar, arterial pressure and who are significantly overweight.

Individuals affected by this unfortunate condition will develop toe numbness, significant loss of feelings in both feet and hands, tingling and burning sensations especially at the end of the day.

Symmetrical presentation of diabetic neuropathy in both feet and both hands is a very important clue for your doctor to be able to identify the exact cause of your symptoms. In case you are experiencing tingling and loss of feeling only in one foot or one hand, the actual culprit for your condition might be of other nature.

In medical history nerve damage due to elevated blood sugar levels is classified into four groups depending on what nerve areas are affected causing the specific symptoms presented in a patient. Autonomic neuropathy significantly affects digestive function leading to bowel, bladder and even sexual problems.

Peripheral neuropathy will cause discomfort in upper and lower extremities, numbness and burning feelings. Focal nerve damage can show up in virtually any area of the body. Finally, proximal type of neuropathy leads to nerve damage in the hip area, namely, buttocks, hips and thighs.

Traditional medicine offers very little support for diabetic patients and resorts to merely managing the symptoms and failing to look deeply into the actual underlying causes of this condition.

Alternative medicine, on the other hand, offers a myriad of natural approaches and remedies to manage both causes and symptoms of the diabetic neuropathy.

Alpha Lipoic acid has been proven to be very effective in managing diabetes and its symptoms. Taking 20 to 50 mg daily is in most cases sufficient in controlling neuropathy especially if initiated at earlier stages of the disease.

Acetyl L-carnitine is another important natural remedy for naturopathy and works by addressing muscle pain and improves mood. If taken at doses of 100 to 300 mgs 3 times per week, it was shown to not cause side effects of over stimulation.

B group vitamins are essential ingredients in any natural treatment of diabetic nerve damage, they additionally support heart function, promote good mood, mental clarity and give you lots of energy naturally.

Ginko Biloba extract has been used in traditional Chinese medicine for centuries and should be included as your treatment for managing pain and discomfort associated with diabetic neuropathy. This traditional supplement significantly improves cognitive function and improves blood circulation.

The most common natural treatments to manage pain that comes hand in hand with nerve damage is acupuncture and massage. Both of these natural techniues will promote a sense of relaxation and well-being triggering the production of endorphins, natural pain killers.

Diet and moderate exercise are one of the most important natural ways to deal with neuropathy along with taking herbs and vitamins. All these factors will bring your blood sugar under control, since poorly controlled blood sugar will cause further deterioration of nerve fibers leading to worsening of your symptoms.

Chapter 10: Neuropathy Therapy Options That Can Keep You Moving

Neuropathy does not have to leave you sitting on the side lines watching life pass you by. Though there might not be a cure for this horrific disease the symptoms and pain are manageable by neuropathy treatments. There are several treatment and therapy options available for patients to take advantage of.

Medications

Common ailments such as a headache or toothache can be treated with simple over the counter medications such as Ibuprofen and aspirin do very little to help relieve the pain caused by severe nerve damage. Medication is needed that can focus on the nerves that are causing pain and treat the symptoms that are felt.

Medication such as: Duloxetine hydrochloride has been given the seal of approval from the F.D.A to treat diabetic neuropathy, antidepressants', Topical cream treatment with capsaicin are just a few of the medications that might be prescribed to help treat the symptoms and pain from neuropathy.

Medications might have side effects so please make sure you are aware if the medication you are taking will leave you feeling drowsy, dizzy, nauseated and could affect your blood pressure.

Injection Therapy

Therapeutic nerve blockers might be another form of neuropathy therapy doctors might encourage suffers to try. By injecting nerve blockers into areas of the body that are experiencing the most pain can provide temporary relief. Injections could consist of steroids that decrease the flare ups, anesthetics and opioids are all forms of nerve blockers that can give a patient temporary relief but nothing long lasting.

Physical Therapy

Might be suggested in order to help restore the range of motions one might have lost or struggle with due to neuropathy in feet that causes numb feet and tingling feet making walking a challenge. Physical therapy will help the patient strengthen muscles that might have grown weak.

Surgery

Surgery as a form of treatment for neuropathy might be one if not your last attempt at seeking pain relief. Very few doctors will treat peripheral neuropathy with surgery but those suffering from carpal tunnel can receive relief from surgery.

Diabetic Neuropathy affects millions of people each year. Though the disorder is complex and no cure has been found there is a new wave of hope for some. A small group of physicians that have been specially trained are able to decompress the nerves through surgery that can relieve some of the pressure a patient with diabetic neuropathy might have.

Neuropathy Support Formula

Neuropathy Support Formula that can be used as a neuropathy treatment and when used daily can produce amazing pain free results. The dynamic combination of vitamin s B1 and B12, herbs and alpha-lipoc acid releases long lasting pain relief from neuropathy pain.

Chapter 11: Reducing Neuropathy The Natural Way

Neuropathy is a disease that has plagued millions of people all over the world. This is a dreadful disease that has haunted a lot of people so much so that several cures and treatments have been painstakingly implored. In fact, a number of pharmaceutical companies have dedicated their research endeavors into finding the best treatment and therapy for neuropathy.

Neuropathy is a condition that denotes the damage of the nerves of the peripheral nervous system. This damage can be attributed to a lot of causes including diseases of the nerves, and side effects of systemic illnesses.

There are basically four patterns of neuropathy which are mononeuropathy, polyneuropathy, mononeuritis multiplex, and autonomic neuropathy. The most common of these is peripheral polyneuropathy.

Peripheral polyneuropathy affects the feet and the legs. Some of the manifestations of this disease include autonomic changes, sensory changes, and varying combinations of weaknesses. While the degree of the manifestations varies from person to person, the symptoms are entirely dependent on some factors.

These factors include motor, sensory, type of nerves affected, and the location of the nerves in the body. Some of the most common symptoms of neuropathy are spasms, cramps, and muscle weakness. In addition, tingling, numbness, and loss of balance may also be experienced.

One of the determined causes of neuropathy is the complication of diabetes. This complication involves both Type 1 and Type 2 diabetes. Thus, most diabetic people are suffering from neuropathy. Although there are a lot of prescribed drugs that are available for the relief and treatment of neuropathy, a lot of people want to patronize natural ways of treating this disease.

One of the natural ways of treating neuropathic pain is taking vitamins and minerals that aid in the treatment or prevention of neuropathy. These include Magnesium, Vitamin B6, Alpha Lipoic

Acid, Vitamin E, and Acetyl-L Carnitine to name a few.

Magnesium is an important nutrient that helps the muscles relax. Moreover, this nutrient is involved in metabolic enzymes such as the communication of nerve signals throughout the body, and in the brain. According to one the testimonies of doctors, neuropathic patients taking Magnesium are showing great improvements.

On the other hand, Vitamin B6 supplementation provides a significant protection against the development of this disease in diabetic patients. It is worth noting that most of the patients with neuropathy are found out to be Vitamin B6 deficient.

Alpha Lipoic Acid has long been used for the treatment and supplementation of diabetes and its complications, neuropathy being one among these. Finally, Vitamin E is proven to improve mild to moderate nerve-type pain. It has also been proven effective for the treatment of neuropathy symptoms.

Chapter 12: Nutrition's Role In Neuropathy

Neuropathy has a wide variety of causes, and nutritional causes are a major subset of it. Neuropathy is typically your first diagnosis when patients complain with symptoms like numbness, pin-and-needle sensation, burning sensations, pain or loss of sensations.

When it affects the nerves supplying the muscles, it may result in weakness of muscle, muscle atrophy, lack of fine muscle control which may result in many symptoms depending on which muscles are affected.

But one cause of peripheral neuropathy that is not readily thought to be associated with neuropathy is food allergy. The association between food allergy and neuropathy is often overlooked because only recently conclusive evidence from research has become available establishing a certain link between neuropathy and allergic response to certain food items.

The most common culprits so far are derivatives of glutamic acid and aspartic acid, gluten, pesticides on fruits and vegetables and food coloring dyes. One very common artificial sweetener, Aspartame, is used in fruit juices, diabetic food and numerous other products, is one of the most commonly recognized allergen triggering symptoms of neuropathy, but this also affects the auditory nerve, causing tinnitus.

Consumption of large ⍰uantities greatly increases the chances of having the neuropathy. Often, stopping the consumption of aspartame cures the symptoms almost entirely.

Many more agents commonly found in food may cause an allergic response which may present as neuropathy. The ones that are currently believed to be responsible for most of the cases are Azino-moto (Mono Sodium Glutamate) which is commonly used in Chinese foods, gluten found in wheat containing edible items, some coloring dyes used in foods.

Not only these, but normal fully natural food items like fruits, eggs, and milk may be the cause of food allergy induced neuropathy. Often it may happen, that the tracking of the allergy causing food item may not be very simple and straightforward.

So what if your neuropathy is suspected to be due to food allergy? The main diagnostic test used is a Radioallergosorbent Test (RAST Test) which detects antibodies against "common" food allergens.

Since not all antigens could be detected in 100% of cases, sometimes the treatment may involve just hit and trial in which suspected food items are stopped for few week and observed whether it alleviates the neuropathy.

Also it would be advisable to stop common known allergens like aspartame, MSG, food dyes, and gluten and observe if the symptoms are alleviated by this. Also thoroughly wash fruits and vegetables before consuming, as pesticides present on them could be the cause.

If you are one of the many thousands of sufferers of Neuropathy, you know all too well that numbness and tinglingis still a pain to deal with.

Peripheral Neuropathy is a condition that is characterized by altered sensation or a change in motor control of a body part. The nerve becomes irritated or damaged and it no longer conducts the messages it should. If your neuropathy is left untreated, it will begin to affect your quality of life.

Chapter 13: Reversing Neuropathy

Neuropathy refers to damage to the peripheral nerves which interferes with the normal functioning of the nerve. Neuropathy can be secondary to another disease or due to direct injury to nerves (trauma, toxins, immune attack, etc). Knowing which neuropathy is reversible and, which is not is of paramount importance.

Many a times there may be a permanent damage to the nerve, and the neuropathy cannot be reversed while sometimes it is fully reversible. The nerve damage may also be intermediate between the two, and there may be some reversal of neuropathy with appropriate treatment.

Neuropathies due to food allergies are often reversible and avoiding the allergy inciting food is the mainstay of therapy. In almost all the cases, the neuropathy is fully reversible and nerve function becomes normal after few weeks of stopping the intake of allergen.

In most of the cases, the neuropathy secondary to adverse effects of a drug is also reversible and stopping the drug or reducing its dose often reverses the neuropathy.

The neuropathy due to Guillain-Barre syndrome is often almost fully reversible with adequate treatment, although full reversal may take up to a year. The main treatment is with immunoglobulin given as intravenous injection and supportive care to prevent any complications.

The neuropathy due to vitamin deficiency is most of the times reversible but there can be also some permanent damage to the nerve and hence a neuropathy that is not fully reversible. The treatment for reversing the neuropathy is replenishment of the deficient vitamin by either oral supplementation or by intramuscular injection.

Neuropathies secondary to other systemic illness may or may not be reversible or sometimes only partially reversible. Diabetes mellitus is a disease in which many different patterns of neuropathy can occur. Some forms of diabetic neuropathies like mononeuropathies (involving only one nerve) and radiculopathies (involving nerve roots) are fully reversible and do not require any specific therapy.

However, one another form, which most often involves lower limbs, is often progressive and irreversible despite treatment. Still tight control of blood-glucose levels should be followed to at least slow the progression and prevent other complications of diabetes.

Hypothyroidism (Myxedema) causes entrapment neuropathies, and majority of these are reversible in the early stages if adequate treatment with thyroid hormone replacement is provided. Other types of entrapment neuropathies like Carpal Tunnel Syndrome are fully reversible in initial stages if treated adequately.

Treatment is providing rest to the wrist, NSAID drugs (like Ibuprofen), or steroid injection in wrist and surgery (done in refractory cases not responding to treatment options). Later there may be some permanent damage, and it may be only partially reversible even with surgical treatment.

Chapter 14: Peripheral Neuropathy Symptoms

Peripheral neuropathy is a widely occurring disease condition, but people usually do not care about peripheral neuropathy symptoms until the condition worsens and the situation is diagnosed to be advanced peripheral neuropathy. The condition shows up in varying degrees of pain and suffering and is commonly found in diabetic patients.

The symptoms peripheral in neuropathy are caused due to damage of the nerves and thus disrupt the nerve signals that connect the spinal cord to the body parts. As the name implies, all the peripheral nerves, the sensory, motor and autonomic nerves are affected due to this.

The nerves in the body work like the electrical wiring system and this is damaged which show up as peripheral neuropathy symptoms. This will often lead to weakness, tingling and pain in the extremities of the feet and hand. The intensity of the neuropathy differs from one person to another with the peripheral neuropathy symptoms being different.

The person inflicted with peripheral neuropathy will find it difficult to manage coordination between the body parts and moving the legs or hands even might become painful. The patient will also be mentally let down due to this condition which makes the person weak and painful. Neuropathy and its symptoms often lead to depression.

People who suffer from symptoms of peripheral in neuropathy are said to experience the feel of wearing socks or gloves when they are not using any of these. This feeling is cause due to a loss of sensation in the feet and the hands. It has been found that this disease condition has been around for years, but Neuropathy symptoms were misdiagnosed with other related disease conditions.

The major complication with this disease condition is that the damage that has been already caused cannot be reversed with any medication and the medicines and home remedies that are available can only be used to prevent further damages.

The first signs of peripheral in neuropathy symptoms have to be recognized by people and diabetic patients should have their feet freꟺuently checked for peripheral neuropathy. In the initial stages, if this condition is diagnosed, it can help to stop a whole lot of possible damage to the body. The patient should also follow proper hygiene and protect the feet from any kind of infection.

In case of an unnoticed wound or infection, the feet will not have any sensation to recognize this wound as a result of peripheral neuropathy symptoms. This when coupled with the prevalent high blood sugar level will worsen the situation.

Chapter 15: How To Manage Neuropathy

Have you ever felt numbness and pain in your feet? A burning sensation on your feet? Then it's a time to consult a doctor. This usually happens in neuropathy. Now the question arises what is neuropathy?

Neuropathy is used to describe the problem with nerves and usually peripheral nerves. Diabetes is the leading cause of neuropathy these days.

Hyperglycaemia affects all the nerves and capillaries of the body and thus neuropathy is often encountered in uncontrolled diabetic condition. Usually, this problem is encountered in old age when the patient usually complains of tingling sensation.

The bad news is that there is no cure for this type of disease. One can only manage, but as there is no permanent treatment for this disease proper management is required. So you need to restrict sugar in your diet. One should not consume sodium aka salt if one wants to diminish the effects of diabetes and neuropathy. Hydration is another important aspect of neuropathy program.

Dietary changes-

The most important change one should bring is a change in his diet. Start your mornings with oatmeal rather than having those sugary cereals. Fruit leathers and homemade fruit snacks are an alternative but one should limit sugar content in his diet.

Exercise daily to fight diabetes-

Start with the simple exercises and then perform pushups on a daily basis to strengthen your cardiovascular system. Brisk walking for 15 minutes is even considered effective when you don't have the habit of regular exercise.

Medication-

Pain relief medicines are available in the market. As there is no permanent cure symptomatic treatment should be given like analgesic for relieving pain. Topical creams are also available in the market for massaging that particular area. Few people even opt for natural treatment for dealing with pain. Neuritis causes extreme pain and it should be treated as soon as possible.

Relax and stay away from stress-

If you stay stressed for long then your body will surely respond to those symptoms in an exaggerated manner thus increasing pain as well. Neuropathy of the hands and neuropathy of feet makes a person dependent on another person for his day to day work as he suffers from extreme pain.

Medicine is necessary, but besides it, a stress-free environment and a happy family are also essential requirements for fighting against this disease. This can be considered as a form of home remedy besides so many other home remedies.

Say no to fried foods and refined sugar

These food items are considered equivalent to poison when consumed in the diabetic state. And plus white carbs even causes harm to a person's body and thus should be avoided as well. With a little precaution, one can live a healthy life with ease. Diabetic pain is sometimes misinterpreted as sciatica pain and thus the proper diagnosis is re?uired to reverse the symptoms.

Chapter 16: Keys To Effective Neuropathy Treatment

Peripheral neuropathy and diabetic neuropathy are both diseases that are brought on by several things. Some of these things are: the nerve damage that occurs with diabetes, the ingestion of toxins over long periods of time, alcohol abuse, genetic diseases, physical trauma and vitamin deficiencies.

While some of these causes can be avoided, there are some (genetic diseases) that cannot be avoided. In those cases, neuropathy treatment is necessary to alleviate the pain and symptoms associated neuropathy.

Eating and Living Healthy

Experts agree that the human body is at its best when it is in peak physical condition. This means that maintaining a healthy weight and eating the right foods can be crucial when battling the effects of neuropathy. What does this mean? It means that the body can fight the symptoms of neuropathy if it is taken care of properly.

Eating a diet rich in antioxidants, omega 3 fatty acids, proteins, green leafy vegetables and low fat foods, can help you maintain a healthy weight, or lose the weight that can complicate diabetic neuropathy. Exercise is also a great way to maintain a healthy lifestyle.

Not only does exercise benefit the body, it also benefits the mind. Exercise can help you keep a positive attitude and outlook, which are both key components to dealing with neuropathy pain.

Avoiding Toxins

Toxins can come in many forms, all of which are harmful in any amount. Some of these toxins include: alcohol, drugs, organic and heavy metals, and excess vitamin B6, which is sometimes given as a remedy for neuropathy.

In most cases, it's easy to avoid ingesting or handling toxins, but sometimes drinking water, old paints and imported goods can be contaminated with toxins. Using a water filter and purchasing certified toxin free imported goods will go a long way to keeping yourself healthy, and fighting the effects of neuropathy.

Pain Management

Managing the pain associated with neuropathy is the most effective neuropathy treatment. Using topical creams with Capsaicin or taking prescription pain medications will help improve your life and keep the pain in check. Some symptoms of neuropathy (numb feet, tingling feet) can also be managed using acupuncture, massage, and heat therapies.

Being diagnosed with neuropathy doesn't mean you have to put aside your life and live with the pain. You can beat neuropathy by taking steps to make sure your neuropathy treatments work effectively.

Chapter 17: Getting Positive About Your Neuropathy Treatment

One of the worst effects of living with peripheral neuropathy and diabetic neuropathy is the toll it takes on your life. Living with the pain of neuropathy can be devastating. Pain in your hands, feet, legs and arms can keep you from living an active and healthy life. So what can you do to strike back at neuropathy and gain back your independence?

Live and think positively- don't let the disease get you down, and here's how.

Get Support

Unfortunately, neuropathy effects more than just the body, it can also effect the mind and spirit. Specialists agree that the constant pain and other associated neuropathy symptoms (tingling feet, numb feet) can be thoroughly discouraging to the sufferer. Pain has the ability to bring about depression, anxiety disorders and other negative personality changes.

Fortunately, there is help, there is hope. One form of effective neuropathy treatment is the encouragement and advice found in support groups. Support groups have been known to help people struggling with all kinds of life problems (drugs, loss, alcohol, weight issues), and people struggling with neuropathy can find solace among others diagnosed with this disease.

Never underestimate the power of positive thinking, encouragement, fellowship with others dealing with the same problems, and the overall happiness found in just getting out and being with other people. You can find support in actual organized support groups, or you can find support among your family and friends.

Get Active

Getting active may seem like a way to increase the pain associated with your neuropathy, but exercise is a great method for neuropathy treatment. Exercise has positive effects across the board. Not only does it keep your body in optimal physical condition, it also helps create a healthy state of mind.

Many active individuals agree that exercise helps to clear the mind and the hormones released during physical activity cause a euphoria that cannot be found in medications.

Exercise alone is a great method for neuropathy treatment, but other methods such as; maintaining a healthy weight, eating healthy foods, staying away from toxins, drinking plenty of water, abstaining from consuming alcohol, and correcting vitamin deficiencies are also great ways to treat neuropathy symptoms.

If these methods of neuropathy treatment fail, using medications (pain blocking injections, topical Capsaicin creams, or prescription medications) are also effective in treating neuropathy pain. Getting your life back from your neuropathy can be as simple as getting support and getting active. Live a positive life despite the negativity of the pain.

Chapter 18: Pain Management And Neuropathy Therapy

Peripheral Neuropathy is a word that describes nerve damage caused by a number of things: diabetes, trauma to nerve cells, toxins such as drugs and alcohol, genetics, vitamin deficiency and the list could go on.

Neuropathy happens when the nerve cells that communicate between the brain and spinal cord get thwarted between various parts of the body resulting in a number of symptoms that can become frustratingly painful.

Areas that could be affected such as a person's internal organs, skin muscles and joints cane set off tingling feet sensations and feelings of numb feet and burning. Patients that have been diagnosed with diabetic neuropathy deal with pain on a daily basis and seek Neuropathy treatment and therapy to help manage the pain.

Pain Management Options

Pain relief and management options vary depending on the approval from their doctor as well as to what extent the neuropathy has affected their muscles and limbs. Options include Physical therapy, Occupational Therapy, Natural therapies, medication as well as injections.

Physical Therapy

Physical therapy can help a patient regain motion and movement to muscles that might have become weekend. Physical therapy will encourage the patient to regain muscle usage and strength by practicing a few daily exercises that can help lessen the pain.

For those who suffer Neuropathy in feet water exercise is a great form of pain management that relinquishes pressure from the feet but will still encourage muscle movement.

Occupational Therapy

Patients diagnosed with neuropathy needs coping skills as they deal with life after diagnosis. Changes will need to be made in regarding their lifestyle and careful thought will need to be had when performing certain everyday activities such as sitting and walking. Occupational therapy will educate the patient on how to position their body to eliminate pain as well walk carefully to prevent falling and hurting themselves further.

Natural Therapy

Natural therapies such as supplementing the body with much needed vitamins and

Alpha -lipoic acid combined with propriety blends can have a calming effect on the nerves and drastically reduce the pain while regenerating the nerves.

Why use therapy at all?

The importance of neuropathy therapy is so that a person suffering from the disease can live their life as normally and positive as possible. Taking away their freedom and forcing them to live with chronic pain limits the joy they are still able to have. With proper neuropathy therapy and treatments most neuropathy patients are able to live independently and actively.

Neuropathy can have a devastating impact on your life. Doctors have developed the most effective treatment to date and if you visit this site, you can ualify for a free sample of this breakthrough nerve support formula.

Chapter 19: How To Get Maximum Benefits From Acupuncture Treatment For Neuropathy

A sound mind resides in a sound body. For the body to be fit, it is essential for a person to get proper rest, exercise regularly, maintain a well-balanced and nutritious diet, get six to eight hours of sleep and keep away from habits like smoking, drinking and eating fast foods.

When a person experiences numbness or weakness in his or her hands, legs or other parts of the body or demonstrates impaired reflexes, this may be a sign of peripheral neuropathy.

Peripheral neuropathy can affect any or all of the nerve groups, including sensory nerves, motor nerves and autonomic nerves. People with peripheral neuropathy may show the following signs:

Numbness and tingling sensations in the hands or feet,

- Acute stabbing pain

- Drop in the blood pressure

- Heaviness in arms and legs

- Weakness of the hands and legs

Causes of Peripheral Neuropathy

Various factors leading to nerve damage are enumerated below-

- Pinched nerves due to herniated disc or muscle spasm

- Glucose intolerance

- Reynaud's disease

- Lupus

- Diabetes

- Kidney disorders

- Hypothyroidism

- Vitamin deficiency, especially of C, B-1, B-6, or B-12

Consulting a neurologist or neurosurgeon who would assess your present health condition and diagnose your nervous disorder would help you get a picture of your prognosis.

Treatment of Peripheral Neuropathy

Before finalizing the right course of treatment for peripheral neuropathy, it is essential to find out the exact cause that has led to this disorder. If it is caused by a vitamin deficiency, then a change in the diet along with vitamin therapy would be helpful.

Likewise, if the nerve damage is due to alcohol abuse or taking a certain medication or toxic substance, then avoiding the substance can restore the health of nerves. One main factor contributing to nerve inflammation is a high sugar and high salt diet.

Even you do not have diabetes, avoiding processed food and sweets will save your nerve function, so that, when you reach 90 years old, you still can walk and think normally.

Alternative Medical therapy for Peripheral Neuropathy

Acupuncture has been found to be highly effective for patients with peripheral neuropathy. Besides the pain relief, patients also experience a marked improvement in nerve conduction after completing the acupuncture course specified by the acupuncturist.

The number of treatments depends on each person's medical condition; for a chronic condition, a few months will be required to recover the nerve function.

Researchers have revealed that electro-acupuncture has helped regenerate nerve cells in rats suffering from spinal cord injuries. There are also human studies that have indicated that acupuncture can bring back the normal sensation of the nerves in the hands and feet.

Furthermore, acupuncture can help the hands regain their strength. If after a nerve injury, you still have developed muscle atrophy after doing physical therapy for a few months, it is the right time to start acupuncture treatment to help the nerves regenerate as soon as possible.

Nervous disorders that acupuncture can correct

Whether it is alcohol, tobacco or junk food addiction, or it is Bell's palsy, dementia, headache or a migraine or stroke, getting acupuncture treatment from a specialist and completing a 12 to 24 course of treatments would provide sufficient blood flow to the nerves.

If diabetes is the major cause of nerve damage, then acupuncture treatment can also prevent a spike in blood sugar level induced by sugar intake and will help stabilize the sugar level in the blood.

Complications of peripheral neuropathy include falls, infection, burns and skin trauma. Besides getting specialized acupuncture treatment, patients should make healthy choices related to their food, exercise and lifestyle. This would help them minimize the risk factors and prevent any further nerve damage, thereby enabling them to enjoy a long and healthy life.

Some of the important things you need to take care are as follows:-

Include fruits, green vegetables, whole grain and protein in your diet for healthy nerves

Exercise 30 minutes-1 hour three times a week to improve the circulation to the peripheral nerves

Avoid smoking or excess drinking, spicy food, exposure to drugs or toxic chemicals.

Chapter 20: Habits And Routines: Powerful Neuropathy Treatment Weapons

Effective neuropathy treatment plans are easier to implement with patients who are able to keep good habits and schedules. It is a well-known fact that our daily habits contribute more to our long-term wellbeing than any other single activity.

What does your daily routine consist of? Are you naturally active, or does it become a challenge for you to motivate yourself? Do you make extra effort to walk more when you park your car to go shopping, for example? How about when performing household or yard tasks?

Our daily habits that affect ourselves includes things like aerobic exercise, drinking soda, tobacco usage, excessive over the counter drug usage, et cetera. It also includes our mental activity; we have the choice to regularly have active mental stimulation such as reading and meditation, versus passive activities such as long periods of watching television.

Unfortunately, most of us never take a hard look at our daily activities, and the impact they're having upon our health. Now, when you're young, these are relatively easy to ignore. But throw in advancing age, and some health challenges, and it becomes a different ballgame.

With chronic pain and neuropathy, sticking to good daily health habits becomes a much more difficult task. But, what I can tell you after taking care of hundreds of patients is that those who have routines and habits fair far better.

Both in terms of physical capacity to enjoy life, and their mental outlook.

One of the reasons for this is more effective neuropathy treatment plans are easier to implement with patients who have good habits and schedules. You can start right now by developing then sticking to a daily routine of your own design. Scheduling and timing of daily things such as meals, light activity, supplements, and even your own self-care goes along way.

One of the reasons this is true is your body has its own biorhythms.

Timing of certain supplements, and even self-treatment throughout the day can make a BIG difference in your outcome. And these are all things your neuropathy treatment specialist is able to assist you with.

Just make sure you engage us and ask for guidance with regard to the most effective neuropathy and chronic pain treatments and activities.

But most importantly ask and learn about the best scheduling, and timing.

Is it possible to cure neuropathy pain naturally and do what you love once again?

The answer is yes, and this practical guide to pain relief will be your first step towards living a painless life.

Inside, you'll find...

What is Neuropathy? How can you help it?

What are the best treatment options for neuropathy

The most common neuropathy symptoms and how you can overcome them.

How to stop neuropathy, prevent damage to nerves, blood vessels eyes and skin.

For neuropathy relief, there are simple foods that you can eat.

What your doctor should do for you to beat neuropathy

This one vitamin will help you keep nerve function normal.

Take only 100mg of this nutrient daily to keep your nerve microcirculation in peak condition.

Two natural and ancient remedies that can help relieve neuropathic discomfort.

Do you want to lower your blood sugar, or worsen your neuropathy? It all depends. Here's how...

How to ease your symptoms in a fraction of the time it takes you watch your favorite sitcom.

Your kitchen cupboard might contain a natural pain reliever.

How to quickly reverse your neuropathy with a simple mineral deficiency

The worrying link between alcohol and neuropathy

How to reduce the strain on your organs and live without neuropathy forever.

Breathing is the best way to reduce your neuropathic symptoms.

How to nourish your nerve cell by eating more of this healthy oil

Touching the right places can increase circulation and help with neuropathy.

You can also learn more about neuropathy!

1

Diabetic neuropathy (also known as diabetes-related neuropathy) is one of the most common side effect of diabetes.

The reason is that diabetes can lead to high blood sugar levels.

2

Finding neuropathy early is the best way to treat it.

3

One of the most common symptoms of neuropathy is constant, recurring or severe pain, especially in the feet and hands. The pain is often described as stabbing or pinpricks, numbness and tingling.

4

You can get neuropathy from diabetes and other conditions, including alcoholism, nutrition deficiencies, infectious diseases such as kidney disease and hormonal problems.

5

Your chances of getting neuropathy can be increased by factors such as age, heredity, malnutrition and the use of medications like taxanes, platinum compounds and vinca alkaloids.

6

You can control neuropathy by controlling your blood sugar. This will prevent any damage to nerves, blood vessels or skin.

7

Neuropathy can be overcome by eating a healthy diet. Get back to eating whole, natural foods. Avoid refined carbs or sugary foods.

8

A complete medical examination is necessary before you can do anything about neuropathy. Do you have an underlying disease?

9

A complete blood test will be done by your doctor to determine the cause of the neuropathy. An EMG (electromyelogram), which measures how well the nerves and muscles work, will be performed by your doctor.

10

One B-100-B-complex vitamin will help to maintain normal nerve function. Do not exceed 200mg daily or take B-6 as high doses could cause neuropathy.

11

To prevent or manage neuropathy, you can also use alpha lipoic Acid. The recommended daily dose is 100mg. This antioxidant maintains the health of your nerve microcirculation.

12

Neuropathy pain can be relieved by reflexology or acupuncture. For faster recovery, Acupuncturists may also recommend Chinese herbs.

13

You don't want your blood sugar to drop too fast, even though it is a great idea. This can increase the intensity of your pain.

14

You can slow down your blood sugar by eating lots of fresh fruits and vegetables, low fat dairy products, whole grains, and other healthy foods.

It is also possible to consume small quantities of beans, fish, chicken, nuts, and poultry.

15

Moving your body is another way to lower blood sugar. It doesn't take long. You can see a huge difference in just 30 minutes per week for 5 days.

16

Capsicin has been used as a pain reliever for centuries. Capsicin can be found in cayenne (also known as red bell pepper). This hot spice can help with neuropathy, surgery recovery, arthritis, and other conditions.

17

For pain relief, oil, creams, or oils with capsaicin can be applied to the affected area. Cayenne pepper works well with foods and can be taken as a supplement in capsules.

18

Magnesium is a vital mineral that your body requires. It uses it to make protein, fatty acids, as well to support nerve function.

19

Studies have shown that people who do not get enough magnesium are more likely to develop neuropathy. It is recommended to consume 400 mg twice daily.

20

In many cases of neuropathy, toxicity plays a critical role. Where is toxicity found? It can get in your body through drugs, alcohol, pesticides or herbicides you ingest or are exposed too.

21

Toxicity is a serious condition that can affect all of your organs, particularly your liver, kidneys and digestive system.

22

Water is a great way to reduce toxicities. As a rule of thumb, you should drink half of your body's weight in ounces per day. For example, if your body weight is 120 pounds, you can drink 60 ounces.

23

Deep breathing is another thing you could do. Do not take just any breath. Breathe deeply and move your belly. You should do at least 100 of these per day.

24

The only way to reverse or manage neuropathy is to reduce toxicity. It is important to address the root cause of neuropathy such as inflammation, viruses, oxidation.

25

Omega 3 fat acids, which are abundant in flaxseed oil and cold water fish, help keep nerve cells healthy. So they are able to transmit nerve signals better.

26

Nettle is a great herb for reducing neuropathy-related inflammation. This herb can lower allergies and hay fever. It may take several weeks to get the results you want, so be patient.

27

Biotin can improve diabetic nervepathy in as little as a month. It is combined with the enzyme, pyruvate carboxylase, to improve neuropathy symptoms.

28

Certain habits can actually worsen neuropathy. One example is smoking. This can reduce blood flow. This can make neuropathy pain worse.

29

Neuropathic pain sufferers can use Message to save their lives. Simply massaging the painful areas, such as the feet or legs, can help relieve the pain by stimulating the nerves.

30

Vitamin B9 can also be called Folic Acid. This vitamin can improve muscle function, and protect your sciatica nerve. The following foods are rich in vitamin B: beans, livers, tomatoes, avocado, and broccoli.

31

Vitamin C works to repair nerve damage and decrease inflammation common among neuropathic sufferers. Take vitamin C-rich foods such as spinach, oranges, cantaloupes, and papayas.

32

Saturated Fat can increase inflammation and worsen neuropathic symptoms. Saturated fats are found in dairy products as well as fatty meats and fried foods. Consider lean alternatives such as soy, fish and lentils. Eat small amounts of healthy oils like vegetable oil, seeds, or nuts.

What is neuropathy and how can it be treated?

Peripheral nervepathy, commonly referred to as neuropathy, can be described as a disorder of the nervous system. This happens when our peripheral nervous system gets damaged.

There are two types, the central nervous and peripheral systems that operate in the human body.

The peripheral nervous network acts as the link between central nervous system (CNS) and all other parts of the body.

These nerves control many organs of the body that we are unable to feel, including heart, lung, stomach and stomach.

The peripheral nerves are responsible for carrying nervous signals from our bodies all the way to our brains through the spinal cords. If one part of this peripheral nervous system is damaged or destroyed, the organs that depend on it will experience immediate malfunctions like feeling pain, inability to function the organ, and so the disorder shall be known as neuropathy.

Types and types of neuropathy

In general, peripheral nervepathy can be classified into two groups: mono-neuropathies as well as poly-neuropathy.

Mono-neuropathies is a form of neuropathy in which only one nerve is affected.

When a type of neuropathy causes damage multiple nerves, it is called poly-neuropathy.

As there are three types, of peripheral nerves within our bodies, we can divide neuropathy into different classes depending on the degree of damage.

1.Sensory neuroscience: Sensory neurons in the body carry nerve signals from our skin, bones, muscles, and brains. We can feel heat, changes in temperature and pain.

Sensory Neuropathy affects our sensory neurons and causes unspeakable pain and other dysfunctions in the organs that are not at risk.

This type of neuropathy usually affects the feet or entire legs.

Sensory neuropathy poses a danger to diabetic patients because they are highly vulnerable against small bleedings and scarring.

Because Sensory Neuropathy prevents diabetic patients from feeling any pain when they get injured while walking barefooted, or from any type of scarring.

Therefore, diabetic patients with Sensory Neuropathy should be extremely cautious when walking or touching other organs.

2.Motor neuropathy is the motor nerves responsible for voluntary movement of our muscles.

These nerves enable our brains direct control of the movement and voluntary muscles.

This type of neuropathy affects the muscles and can lead to muscle weakness, pain cramps, muscle shrinkage, or even muscle death.

Motor neuropathy, which is a condition that affects our main operative muscles and prevents them working properly, can always be irritating.

If left untreated, it can cause permanent injury to the muscle.

3.Autonomic neuralpathy: The autonomic nerves link our brains to our internal organs.

These nerves have a crucial role as our brains control involuntary movements of the internal organs.

Autonomic Neuropathy can also cause severe damage to internal organs, such as the bladder or stomach.

This type can cause severe diseases such as gastroparesis (food can't move through your digestive system properly), irregular heartbeats, impotence, and other serious illnesses.

The most serious and difficult-to-treat form of neuropathy among the three is autonomic.

Causes:

We already know of three types of neuropathy.

There are over a hundred different types of neuropathy. Every one has its own cause.

I tried to concentrate on the most important causes.

*Autonomic nervepathy (such kidney damage) can be caused by systemic diseases such as diabetes, irregular circulation, and other conditions.

*Nerve injuries or trauma are the most common cause of nerve damage.

There are two types of trauma that can lead to neuropathy.

Sudden trauma may be caused by accidents or sports injuries.

This type can be easily treated using surgical techniques.

A daily job that is difficult or too heavy can cause neuropathy.

This type neuropathy requires long-term rest and physiotherapy in order to be treated.

*Breathing problems reduce the oxygen supply to peripheral nerves and can lead to neuropathy.

Nerve damage can also occur from cancers, infections, and autoimmune disorders.

*Intoxication from toxins or excessive alcohol consumption can cause neuropathy.

*Neuromas may be tumors caused by the overgrowth nerve tissue. This can lead to severe neuropathy.

*Smoking can cause disruption to oxygen supply to our nervous systems, and its toxic components can cause serious neuropathy.

Symptoms:

Each type of neuropathy presents with different symptoms.

The most common signs and symptoms of neuropathy include:

*Tingling in legs and hands.

*Losing control in muscles and diseases such as diarrhea and excessive sweating.

*Skin feels tightened and dry.

*Shorp pains in the muscles and bones.

*Muscle weakness, heavy feelings in muscles.

*Internal diseases, such as kidney damage or irregular heartbeat.

*Low blood pressure

*Sexual dysfunction - mainly for men

*Lack of sensations within particular organs.

*Exercising muscles to stretch.

Treatment:

Neuropathy can be treated by surgery, long term physiotherapy or medications.

There are some natural treatments to prevent or treat neuropathy.

*Managing blood sugar and eating a healthy diet are important for diabetic patients.

*Resist the temptation to drink alcohol or get into toxic situations.

*Exercise daily to eliminate muscle cramps.

*Chiropractic massage may be helpful in removing neuropathy.

*Herbs with Alpha Lipid Acid, Vitamin B6, and Cayenne Massage on the Skin can be very helpful. A popular east Asian treatment for neuropathy includes herbal remedies.

*Returning to a healthy food digestion cycle is possible by taking digestive enzymes three days a day.

NEUROPATHY - WHAT IS IT?

Neuropathy can be defined as a condition that causes nerve malfunctions. This could be caused by nerve damage, or another cause.

diseases. Because nerves coordinate the activities of the body, they are crucial. These activities cover all of the body's voluntary and involuntary processes.

You can monitor your breathing rate, heartbeat rate (heartbeat), blood pressure and blood pressure as well as your sexual response, digestion, temperature, and other bodily functions. It allows the body adapt and respond.

Any changes in the body or sytem. If neuropathy is diagnosed, it can affect one or more of the following processes.

NEUROPATHY STYLES

There are many types and varieties of neuropathy. However, the last two are the most prevalent.

Most often acquired by individuals.

Focal Neuropathy refers a specific or group of neuropathies.

A single nerve may only affect one limb. Most often, it affects only the wrist, thigh, or foot. It can cause numbness.

Bell's palsy, paralysis on one or both sides of the face, pain around the chest, double vision, Bell's Palsy and pain in the area surrounding the chest are some common causes. Direct causes are the most common.

Trauma, cold and burns, radiation, tumors and blockage of the blood. Diabetes is known as mononeuropathy.

Cranial Neuropathy can occur when the nerves within the brain or brainstem get damaged. The nerves affected will be affected.

muscles of the eyes and face. Cranial Neuropathy, itself, can be classified into five types.

1. Bell's palsy

The condition occurs when the muscles of one side are paralyzed and become weak. This happens because of trauma.

The seventh cranial nervous system.

2. Microvascular Cranial Nerve Palsy

These conditions affect the nerves within the eyes. It is possible for some muscles to not be moved because the blood flowing through the nerves in the head is blocked. If this happens, you should seek immediate medical assistance.

The person will have double vision.

3. Oculomotor or Third Nerve Palsy

It occurs when the 3rd cranial nerve becomes damaged. This nerve controls pupil constriction and eye movement. This nerve is responsible for controlling pupil constriction and movement in the eyes.

The pupil will not respond to light, and will struggle to control the movement of his eyes. Each eye will be in an outward or downward position.

4. Trochlear Nerve Palsy (or Fourth Nerve Palsy)

This is caused by the weakness of the superior oblique muscular, which can lead to a weakening.

Eye alignment can be caused by misalignment, whether it is in vertical, horizontal or torsional positions. It can affect both one or both eyes. When this happens, the person will tilt his head.

looking.

5. Abducens Palsy/the Sixth Nerve Palsy

This is due to a malfunction of the lateralrectus muscular. It causes the eye to move inward toward the nose. This is most often due to stroke, trauma and viral illness.

Inflammation can also cause infection. It can also develop during birth.

Autonomic Neuropathy (also known as nerve damage) is caused by nerve damage.

For involuntary function such as blood pressure or heart rate, sweating and bowel movements, etc. The symptoms include dizziness and nausea when standing, as well as vomiting after eating. The symptoms may also include dizziness while standing and vomiting when eating.

There may be disturbances in bladder control, bowel movement, and sexual function.

Peripheral Neuropathy represents the most common type. It is caused by damage to peripheral nerves. This causes weakness, numbness and sometimes pain in the.

Both hands and feet. The peripheral nervous systems is responsible for communicating information from the brain to the rest of your body. It is the one that tells the body how it should behave.

The body's internal and external changes will be reflected in your responses. Affected by this type disease, you might feel burns as he cannot feel the temperature changes or pain.

You may have to be careful about what you do with certain areas. It can lead to infection because one won't be able to see which part was injured.

NEUROPATHY CAUSES

There are many types of Althoug Neuropathy.

Yet, it is very similar. There are many possible causes for the disease. Here are a few examples.

1. Heavy Drinking

Alchoholics are generally poor eaters.

Poor diet choices are the cause of vitamin deficiency. This causes nerve damage.

2. Autoimmune disorders

One example of such diseases is lupos. This

Diseases can severely affect the nerves.

3. Diabetes

According to statistics, nearly half of all people have neuropathy associated with diabetes. This is also known as diabetic neuralgia. These people are known as diabetic neuropathy.

High blood pressure, advanced age and being diabetic for a prolonged period increase the likelihood of developing this type of illness.

4. Toxic Substances

People who are exposed too toxic substances like heavy Metals

Most likely, they will have their nerves damaged by chemical agents.

5. Medical Treatment

Certain medications and medicines may cause nerve cell damage. One example of medication that can injure nerve cells is chemotherapy. This is used to treat cancer.

6. Infections

Lhyme disease. Shingles, Epsteinbarr virus. Hepatitis C. leprosy.

Diphteria as well as HIV are examples of viral or bacterial infections that can cause nerve damage.

7. Genetic disorders

Friedreich's disease and Charcot Marie-Tooth syndrome are examples. These disorders may affect the nerve.

functions.

8. Trauma and Injury

Sports injuries, as well as accidents in vehicles, can cause damage to the peripheral nervous systems.

9. Tumors

Both malignant or non-cancerous tumors can grow within the body and eventually press the nerves.

10. Vitamins lacking

B-1, B-6, B-12, vitamin E and Niacin are important.

nerve's health. Deficiency of any one of these vitamins could lead to nerve damage.

11. Bone marrow disorder

There are three main factors that can contribute to the development of neuropathy: bone cancer, lymphoma or amyloidosis.

HOW TO GET RID OFF NEUROPATHY

Neuropathy can be treated by managing the medical conditions, such as diabetes and medications for rheumatoid arthritis. You should have the

Good nutrition is key. It is important to make good choices when choosing what foods to eat. It is possible to effectively eat fruits, vegetables whole grain, lean protein, and whole grains.

Exercise regularly to improve your nervous systems. It is recommended that you exercise regularly, according to doctors.

How to recognize peripheral neuropathy symptoms

Perimeter neuropathy can cause severe pain, particularly for people who have never experienced it before. It can be frustrating and overwhelming to try to adjust to a life with so much pain.

Peripheral Neuropathy symptoms can have a major impact on the quality of life for people with this condition. To make the condition less severe, it's important to understand the causes of the condition and how treatment can be applied.

While peripheral neuropathy is a condition that worsens over time, there are cases where treatment can be helpful.

What then is peripheral nervepathy?

This is a condition that results from nerve damage in the legs, feet fingers, and hands. You can inherit it, but it may also be caused by other factors. The peripheral nerves transmit messages from brain, central nervous system and spinal cord to other body areas.

The damage to the peripheral nerves can make it difficult for people to send and get massages. This can lead many complications.

Different medical conditions can indicate the condition.

It often involves the motor and autonomic nervous systems, as well the sensory nerves.

Although it can affect the peripheral nerves, it can also affect other nervous systems.

Peripheral neuropathy is more common among diabetics.

Types and types of peripheral neuropathy

Two types of neuropathy are common:

Acute neuropathy

It is most often caused by certain illnesses, like diabetes. It takes a very short time for the victim to heal.

Chronic neuropathy

It develops slowly and the symptoms stay the same.

Causes of peripheral Neuropathy

These are some of the many instances where peripheral neuropathy could occur. These are just a few of the more common cases.

Injury

Nerve damage is possible from accidents or sports injuries. These damages can be either minor or major enough to result in the loss of a whole nerve.

Diseases

It can also be caused by certain diseases, including those that affect our endocrine systems like diabetes. Half of those with diabetes suffer from peripheral neuropathy.

Kidney and liver diseases

Perimeter neuropathy is a condition where there's too much toxin.

Hormonal changes

Nerve pains can result from changes in hormones. The proper functioning of the body is dependent on its hormones.

Nerve related issues can also arise from a reduction in thyroxin.

Furthermore, growth hormones can cause bones to grow in excess, leading to more bone fractures and nerve damage.

Alcoholism

A condition known as alcohol neuropathy can also be caused by excessive drinking of alcohol.

Genetics

Some cases of peripheral neuropathy develop while a person is still an infant. Others can develop it during adolescence.

Signs and symptoms of peripheral neuropathy

The symptoms are usually different for each person. But, some people do not show any symptoms. For you to know if you have the disorder or not, it is crucial to consult a doctor.

These symptoms are felt in many parts of the body, including the feet, arms, legs, feet, hands and feet.

Tingling and numbness

People affected often feel "pins and pins" for a time. These symptoms are caused by an improper functioning of nerves.

Loss of Balance

People suffering from the disorder often lose their balance. This is because there is a lack in coordination in different parts.

Hypersensitivity

Even the smallest touch can result in increased sensation for the individual affected

Sensitivity in fingers, feet, and other parts of the body is lost.

Incapability of identifying between hot/cold

Burning sensations and shooting pains. This is more common during the night.

In more severe cases, it can lead to infection, gangrene or foot and/or leg ulcers.

Increased or decreased pain in the skin, or inability to feel pain

Remedies for peripheral neuropathy

While there is no cure, lifestyle changes are a good way to manage the condition. Here are some treatments for peripheral neuropathy.

Alpha lipoic acids

You can find the treatment at most medical clinics. It is an important fatty acid found in most body cells. In the following ways, alpha lipoic Acid can ease peripheral neuropathy.

It's a great help in energy production

Additionally, it aids in body function

It works as an antioxidant and helps to eliminate any harmful free radicals

converts blood sugar into energy

Magnesium

Studies show that people can have difficulty getting enough magnesium from their diets. Magnesium deficiency is a common problem. Magnesium, an important mineral in the formation fatty acid, is essential.

It helps blood clot and creates new cells. When magnesium deficiency is present, peripheral neuropathy symptoms are worse.

Magnesium supplements can be purchased at your local pharmacy. The following are other sources of magnesium

Legumes

Sunflower seeds

Nuts

Green vegetables

Seafood

Cayenne pepper

It's a great ingredient for spicing foods and also has medical benefits. Capsaicin, which is a chemical component found in cayenne pepper, can provide natural pain relief as well as aiding in digestion.

It's also an effective treatment for those suffering from peripheral nerve damage. It can also be added to a diet.

Exercise

Exercise is a key part of your overall health. It can also be used to relieve pain.

Regular exercise will improve blood flow to the areas most affected by peripheral nervepathy. This includes the hands, fingers, and legs. Exercise can nourish damaged nerves by stimulating them.

It is not necessary to exercise a lot. It can be helpful to have a walking plan or a job that you do every morning.

www.ingramcontent.com/pod-product-compliance
Lightning Source LLC
Chambersburg PA
CBHW060234030426
42335CB00014B/1456